Cookbook for Leukemia Diet:

A detailed cookbook for Leukemia

By

Crystal M. Thompson

DISCLAIMER PAGE

Table of Content

DISCLAIMER PAGE

Table of Content

CHAPTER 1

CHAPTER 2

CHAPTER 3

CHAPTER 4

CHAPTER 5

CHAPTER 1

Leukemia is a blood malignancy that affects the bone marrow. It is distinguished by the excessive proliferation of aberrant white blood cells in the bone marrow, which drive out good blood cells. This may result in a variety of symptoms and problems.

Leukemia Types:

There are four major varieties of leukemia, which are further classified as acute or chronic:

1. Acute Lymphoblastic Leukemia (ALL):This kind of leukemia is more frequent in youngsters and particularly attacks lymphoid cells.

2. Acute Myeloid Leukemia (AML): AML is a kind of leukemia that affects myeloid cells and may affect both children and adults. It tends to move quickly.

3. Chronic Lymphocytic Leukemia (CLL): CLL is a kind of leukemia that predominantly affects B lymphocytes and is most usually diagnosed in adults, particularly those over the age of 50.

4. Chronic Myeloid Leukemia (CML): CML is a kind of leukemia that affects myeloid cells and typically advances slowly, with a chronic phase that

may later transition into an accelerated or blast crisis phase.

Leukemia Symptoms:

Fatigue, pale complexion, easy bruising or bleeding, frequent infections, unexplained weight loss, enlarged lymph nodes, bone or joint pain, stomach discomfort, night sweats, and trouble breathing are all common signs of leukemia.

Diagnosis and Therapy:

Blood tests, bone marrow aspiration and biopsy, and occasionally imaging examinations are used to diagnose leukemia. Depending on the kind and stage of leukemia, treatment options may include chemotherapy, radiation therapy, targeted therapy, immunotherapy, and stem cell transplantation. Treatment strategies are adapted to each individual's unique situation.

Prognosis:

Survival rates for leukemia vary according to kind, stage of diagnosis, patient age, and other variables. Treatment advances have improved results for many leukemia patients, with certain kinds of illness curing at a high rate.

CHAPTER 2

A well-balanced and nutritious diet is critical to the general health and well-being of people with leukemia. A leukemia diet should include needed nutrients, immune system support, weight maintenance, and management of any adverse effects of the illness and its therapies. Remember that dietary advice may differ based on the kind and stage of leukemia, as well as the individual's health situation and treatment strategy. It is critical to get tailored advice from a healthcare practitioner or qualified dietician. Here are some basic dietary recommendations for people with leukemia:

1. Balanced Diet: To guarantee a broad range of
nutrients, aim for a well-balanced diet that contains
a variety of foods from all food categories.

2. Adequate Calories: Maintaining a healthy weight
requires consuming enough calories to fulfill your
energy requirements. Consider calorie-dense meals
like avocados, almonds, and full-fat dairy items if
you're suffering unexpected weight loss.

3. Protein is essential for cell repair and
immunological function. Include lean protein
sources in your diet, such as fowl, fish, beans,
lentils, tofu, and dairy products.

4. Fruits and Vegetables: To acquire critical vitamins, minerals, and antioxidants, eat a range of colorful fruits and vegetables. These nutrients may aid with immune system support.

5. Whole Grains: Whole grains, such as brown rice, quinoa, whole wheat bread, and oats, include fiber, which improves digestion.

6. Healthy Fats: For general health, include sources of healthy fats in your diet such as avocados, nuts, seeds, and olive oil.

7. Hydration: Drink lots of water throughout the day to stay hydrated.

Fluid intake may also be increased by drinking clear broths, herbal teas, and diluted fruit juices.

8. Small, Frequent Meals: If you have a low appetite or energy level, eating smaller, more frequent meals may be simpler to handle.

9. Limit Processed Foods: Reduce your intake of processed and sugary foods, which have little nutritional value and may damage your immune system.

10. Soft Foods: If you have mouth sores or trouble swallowing, choose soft and easy-to-chew foods such as mashed potatoes, yogurt, and smoothies.

11. Food Safety: To limit the risk of infection, practice good food safety. Avoid eating raw or undercooked meals, and thoroughly wash all fruits and vegetables.

12. Supplements: Your healthcare professional may offer supplements such as vitamin D, iron, or others to treat particular deficiencies based on your unique requirements.

13. Dietary limitations: If you have special dietary limitations or concerns, talk to your healthcare team or a nutritionist to make sure your diet is in line with your treatment plan.

14. Be Informed: Be aware of any possible
interactions between your food and any drugs or
treatments you're getting. In this respect, your
healthcare team may advise you.

Remember that dietary recommendations for
leukemia patients might vary depending on
individual characteristics, and they may need to be
altered over time as treatment advances and side
effects change. Always collaborate with your
healthcare team to develop a food plan that matches
your unique requirements while also supporting
your overall health throughout your leukemia
journey.

CHAPTER 3

While there are no cookbooks specifically designed for leukemia, people with the disease may benefit from cookbooks that concentrate on cancer-friendly or cancer-supportive diets. These cookbooks often include recipes and dietary advice that may assist patients in meeting their nutritional requirements while also managing the adverse effects of cancer and its therapies.

Consult a Registered Dietitian: Working with a registered dietitian who specializes in cancer nutrition is one of the greatest methods to build a tailored leukemia diet plan. They may provide personalized recommendations, meal plans, and recipes based on a person's unique requirements, treatment plan, and dietary preferences.

When using cookbooks or online resources, keep in mind the specific dietary recommendations provided by the healthcare team, as the dietary needs of people with leukemia can vary greatly depending on factors like the type of leukemia, treatment plan, and any existing nutritional deficiencies. Consult a healthcare practitioner or a dietician to confirm that dietary choices are appropriate for the individual's unique condition and treatment objectives.

Keep in mind that the major purpose of a leukemia diet is to promote general health, provide enough nourishment, and aid in the management of the side effects of leukemia and its therapies.

Symptoms of Leukemia

Leukemia is a blood malignancy that affects the bone marrow. Leukemia symptoms vary based on the kind of leukemia, its stage, and individual circumstances. Common leukemia symptoms include:

1. tiredness: A typical symptom of leukemia is persistent and inexplicable tiredness. It is often severe and incapacitating.

2. Pale Skin: Anemia, caused by a reduction in healthy red blood cells, may cause pale skin and widespread weakness.

3. Easy Bruising and Bleeding: Because leukemia reduces platelets (thrombocytopenia), it may cause easy bruising, nosebleeds, and prolonged bleeding from minor wounds or bruises.

4. Frequent Infections: Because leukemia often damages white blood cells, it weakens the immune system and makes people more prone to infections. illnesses that reoccur, such as fever, sore throat, or respiratory illnesses, might be a warning indication.

5. Unexplained Weight Loss: In certain leukemia instances, significant and unexplained weight loss might occur.

6. Swollen Lymph Nodes: Swollen lymph nodes, especially in the neck, armpits, or groin, may indicate leukemia.

7. Bone and Joint Pain: Some persons with leukemia feel bone pain, joint pain, or arm and leg discomfort.

8. Abdominal pain: An enlarged spleen or liver (hepatosplenomegaly) may induce abdominal pain or a sense of fullness.

9. Night Sweats: Unrelated to room temperature or exertion, night sweats may be an indication of leukemia.

10. Breathing Issues: Leukemia may cause shortness of breath and difficulty breathing in certain people.

11. Swollen Gums and Frequent Nosebleeds: Gum swelling and bleeding may occur as a result of leukemia. This is more prevalent in patients with acute leukemia.

12. CNS Symptoms: Leukemia cells may infiltrate the central nervous system (CNS) and produce symptoms such as headaches, impaired vision, or disorientation in rare circumstances.

It is crucial to remember that these symptoms are not limited to leukemia and may be caused by a variety of different medical problems. However, if you or someone you know is having chronic or inexplicable symptoms, it is critical to get medical assistance as soon as possible. Early detection and treatment are critical for controlling leukemia and increasing the likelihood of a favorable result.

If leukemia is suspected, a number of procedures, including blood testing and bone marrow biopsies, will be performed to confirm the diagnosis and define the type and stage of leukemia.

CHAPTER 4

Risk

Leukemia is a complicated illness with many unknown origins. Several risk factors, however, have been found that may enhance an individual's chances of acquiring leukemia. It's crucial to remember that having one or more risk factors does not ensure that you'll get leukemia, and many individuals with leukemia have no known risk factors. Here are some of the most prevalent risk factors for leukemia:

1. Age: Although leukemia may develop at any age, it is more frequent in older people.

2. Gender: There is a modest gender bias in certain kinds of leukemia.

AML, for example, is somewhat more frequent in males than in women, although CLL is more prevalent in men.

3. Radiation Exposure: Excessive ionizing radiation exposure, such as that encountered by survivors of nuclear accidents or atomic bomb blasts, has been linked to an increased risk of leukemia. Radiation therapy used in medical treatments may also raise the risk, although the advantages of treatment usually exceed the hazards.

4. Chemical Exposure: Exposure to certain chemicals prevalent in certain jobs and industrial settings, such as benzene and formaldehyde, has been associated with an elevated risk of leukemia. Furthermore, chemotherapy medications used to treat other malignancies may raise the likelihood of acquiring leukemia as a secondary malignancy.

5. Genetic Factors: Certain genetic disorders, such as Down syndrome, Bloom syndrome, and Fanconi anemia, are linked to an increased chance of developing leukemia.

6. Family History: While most instances of leukemia are not inherited, having a close relative (parent or sibling) with leukemia may raise the risk somewhat.

7. Previous Cancer Treatment: People who have previously had certain cancer therapies, such as radiation therapy or chemotherapy, are more likely to develop leukemia as a consequence of the treatment.

8. Blood Disorders: Precursors to leukemia, such as myelodysplastic syndromes (MDS), might increase the chance of developing AML.

9. Viral Infections: Exposure to viruses such as the human T-cell leukemia virus (HTLV-1) has been linked to an elevated risk of acquiring certain kinds of leukemia in certain situations.

10. Smoking: Tobacco use is associated with an increased risk of developing AML, especially in adults.

It is crucial to highlight that the majority of occurrences of leukemia occur in people who have no known risk factors, and having one or more risk factors does not ensure the disease's development.

Furthermore, continuing research is always revealing new knowledge regarding the causes and risk factors for leukemia. If you are concerned about your risk of having leukemia or have a family history of the illness, it is best to consult with a healthcare specialist who can give information and, if required, undertake proper testing.

CHAPTER 5

Survival

The kind of leukemia, the stage at diagnosis, the individual's age and general condition, and the exact therapy administered may all have a significant impact on survival rates. Survival rates are often presented as percentages and are based on data from large groups of individuals who have the same form of leukemia. It should be noted that these figures are just approximations and do not indicate the prognosis of any person with leukemia. Survival rates vary over time as treatment choices and results improve. Here are some general survival rates for several forms of leukemia:

1. ALL (Acute Lymphoblastic Leukemia):

- Pediatric ALL: Over the years, the survival rate for children with ALL has increased dramatically. Today, the 5-year survival rate for pediatric ALL is above 90%, and with adequate therapy, many children may be cured.

- Adult ALL: Adults with ALL have a worse 5-year survival rate than children, often ranging from 30% to 50%. However, results might vary depending on criteria like as age, ALL subtype, and response to therapy.

2. AML (Acute Myeloid Leukemia):

- The 5-year survival rate for AML varies based on age and unique genetic alterations. Adults with AML have a 5-year survival rate of roughly 20-30%.

- Younger persons and those who can withstand rigorous therapies such as stem cell transplantation have a better chance of survival.

3. CLL (Chronic Lymphocytic Leukemia):
- Because CLL is a slow-progressing leukemia, many patients may not need urgent therapy.
- CLL has a good 5-year survival rate, frequently reaching 85%.
- Treatment choices are often influenced by an individual's general health, illness progression, and other circumstances.

4. CML (Chronic Myeloid Leukemia):
- The introduction of targeted medicines such as tyrosine kinase inhibitors (TKIs) has resulted in considerable improvements in treatment results for CML.

- For individuals getting proper therapy, the 5-year survival rate for CML is high, generally reaching 90%.

It is critical to underline that leukemia is a very curable malignancy, and breakthroughs in treatment choices have resulted in better results for many people. As new cures are discovered and established treatments grow more effective, survival rates continue to rise. Furthermore, each person's experience with leukemia is unique, and variables other than statistics, such as treatment response and general health, have a considerable influence in deciding their prognosis.

If you or someone you love has been diagnosed with leukemia, it is critical to speak with an oncology-focused healthcare team to build a tailored treatment plan and understand the individual's prognosis and anticipated results.

Cancer diet during chemotherapy

Making wise dietary choices can aid your immune system's battle against cancer. The meals you consume during active cancer treatment will depend on any adverse effects you are experiencing. Learn how to use nutrition to manage side effects.

Overall, choose foods that offer you adequate calories (to maintain your weight), protein (to help repair tissues damaged by cancer therapy), nutrients such as vitamins and minerals, and water (necessary for your body's functioning). Exercise may also assist with treatment-related hunger and digestive difficulties.